Title

Unlock Your Strength:

Build the Body You Love at Home

Copyright

All rights reserved. No part of this publication may be reproduced, distributed, or transmitted in any form or by any means, including photocopying, recording, or other electronic or mechanical methods, without the prior written permission of the publisher, except in the case of brief quotations embodied in critical reviews and certain other noncommercial uses permitted by copyright law.

Copyright © (Peterson Caleb), (2024).

Introduction

Open Your Solidarity: Assemble the Body You Love at Home

Fed up with feeling threatened by the rec center? Prepared to jettison the costly enrollments and swarmed storage rooms?

Unlock Your Strength is your enabling manual for building the body you love, **all from the solace of your own home**. This far reaching program goes past fundamental bodyweight works out, offering available yet viable schedules that use regular items and insignificant hardware. Whether you're a finished fledgling or a wellness devotee searching for a new test, this book gives all that you want to:

*Open your potential:** Find a customized way to deal with wellness that spotlights on developing fortitude, further developing adaptability, and supporting your certainty. *Embrace convenience:** No more reasons! Plan productive exercises around your bustling timetable, utilizing promptly accessible things like seats, water containers, and, surprisingly, your own body weight. **Challenge yourself:** Progress through an assortment of activity programs customized to various

wellness levels and objectives, guaranteeing you're continually invigorated and spurred.
*Create solid habits:** Gain significant experiences into sustenance, rest, and stress the executives, making an all encompassing way to deal with your prosperity.
*Praise your success:** Keep tabs on your development with inspirational instruments and direction, permitting you to observe your change and embrace a better, more joyful you.

Disregard the restrictions of traditional rec centers and open your actual expected in the natural space of your home. With

Unlock Your Strength, you'll acquire the information, devices, and motivation to shape your body, support your energy, and open a freshly discovered feeling of strengthening - all in your own specific manner.

Is it true or not that you are prepared to set out on your excursion to a more grounded, better you? Begin opening your solidarity today!

Table of contents

Adapting to lifestyle changes
changes
Tracking progress
Overcoming challenges

Mindset and goal setting

When it comes to achieving your dream physique without going to the gym, it is critical to create the right attitude and outline prospective objectives. Following that, we will look at a few key issues:

. Maintain a positive mindset towards your body and overall well-being.
   - Based on assurance and confirmation, appreciate your body for what it is while working towards growth.

. **Realistic Expectations:** - Set achievable and realistic wellness goals based on your current level of affluence.
   - Value improvements need effort, and progress may take many forms.

Long-Term Perspective:** - Focus on your long-term prosperity cycle rather than seeking helpful strategies.
   - See how smart improvements lead to successful outcomes.

. **Embrace the Process:** - Participate in the excursion and appreciate little accomplishments along the way.
   - Shift your focus from immediate results to good patterns and improvements you're making.

 Adaptability: - Be flexible and willing to change your goals as your collaboration grows.
   - Life is changing, and your goals may need a shift in how you approach pushing situations.

. **Intrinsic Motivation:** - Identify internal sources of inspiration, such as increased energy, improved mood, or involvement in daily activities.
   - Encourage a shine for the course of mindfulness rather than relying only on outside funding.

Goal Specificity: - Clearly define prosperity targets, such as strength, adaptability, perseverance, or bodily game plan.
   - Divide more significant goals into smaller, more manageable accomplishments for pride.

Continuous Learning: - Prioritise prosperity cooperation as a valuable development opportunity.
   - Stay up to date on different action tactics, culinary strategies, and generally successful rehearsals.

** Develop resilience by adapting to disasters and taking preventative measures.
   - View impacts as opportunities to learn and grow, rather than reasons to give up.

 Enjoy the Process: - Find delight in the workouts you choose for prosperity, such as moving, climbing, or practicing yoga.
   - Make your workouts enjoyable in order to stay focused on long-term commitments.

 Self-Reflection: - Consistently review your actions and goals.

- Understand the aspects that contribute to progress or difficulty, and alter your methods accordingly.

By promoting a positive attitude and defining realistic, comprehensive objectives, you provide the groundwork for a reasonable and fulfilling wellness experience tailored to your preferences and goals.

Home workout and equipment

Making astounding home activities without the requirement for expensive gear isn't just reasonable yet additionally open. Here are a few clues and thoughts:

 Bodyweight Exercises: - Consolidate fundamental bodyweight practices including squats, jumps, push-ups, and boards.

- Progress to additional perplexing variations as your solidarity and perseverance increment.

HIIT (Focused energy Span Training): - Plan focused energy stretch exercises that blend explosions of extraordinary practice in with brief recuperation spans.
- Models incorporate hopping jacks, burpees, and hikers.

Resistance Bands: - Put resources into obstruction groups for expanded opposition during exercises like bicep twists, horizontal raises, and leg press.
- Groups are versatile, convenient, and appropriate for all exercise levels.

Dumbbells or Family Items:
   - Use free weights if accessible, or be innovative with family things like water bottles, rucksacks loaded down with books, or jars.
   - Adjust exercises, for example, hand weight squats, above presses, and columns.

 Yoga Mat: - A comfortable yoga mat is vital for floor activities and extending.
   - Use it for exercises like sit-ups, boards, and yoga extends.

Stability Ball: - Integrate a steadiness ball for center activities and equilibrium preparing.

- Practices like solidness ball crunches and spans work various muscle gatherings.

 Jump Rope: - Incorporate a leap rope for an incredible cardiovascular activity.
   - Working out with rope further develops coordination and consumes calories.

 Step Platform: - Utilize a stage for vigorous schedules including step-ups, bounces, and rushes.
   - Change the level for evolving power.

Sliders: - Slide circles or furniture sliders might expand trouble to exercises like hikers,

rushes, and stomach muscle rollouts.
   - Place them underneath your feet or hands to make a sliding impression.

Online practice Resources: - Investigate online stages and applications giving home activity programs.
   - Follow directed meetings for variety and support.

Circuit Training: - Make circuit-style exercises by blending different practices in with restricted break between sets.
   - This technique keeps up with the pulse up for cardiovascular benefits.

Adaptability: - Adjust exercises relying upon your wellness level and any actual limitations.
   - Steadily increment force and intricacy as you settle in.

Keep in mind, the key is to be predictable and partake simultaneously. Tailor your home activities as you would prefer and dynamically propel yourself. With a tad bit of creative mind, you might accomplish extraordinary outcomes without the requirement for an intricate rec center hardware.

Nutrition for body transformation

Sustenance assumes an essential part in any body change venture. Here are key contemplations for building your fantasy body without heading out to the rec center:

 Caloric Balance:
   - Figure out your day to day caloric necessities in light of your objectives (weight reduction, support, or muscle gain).
   - Make a feasible calorie shortfall for fat misfortune or an excess for muscle building.

Macronutrient Distribution:
   - Balance your admission of macronutrients - proteins, starches, and fats.

- Protein is fundamental for muscle fix and development, starches for energy, and fats for by and large wellbeing.

Whole Food varieties and Supplement Density:
   - Focus on entire, supplement thick food varieties like organic products, vegetables, lean proteins, entire grains, and solid fats.
   - These food varieties give fundamental nutrients, minerals, and fiber.

Meal Timing:
   - Consider spreading your feasts over the course of the day to keep up with energy levels and backing digestion.
   - Incorporate pre-and post-exercise sustenance for ideal execution and recuperation.

Hydration:
   - Remain satisfactorily hydrated as water is fundamental for different physical processes, including absorption and digestion.

- Go for the gold 8 glasses of water each day, changing in light of individual requirements and action level.

Portion Control:
    - Be aware of piece sizes to abstain from indulging.
    - Utilize more modest plates and pay attention to your body's yearning and completion signals.

. **Limit Handled Foods:**
    - Limit admission of handled and sweet food sources.
    - These can add to overabundance calorie utilization and may come up short on supplements.

 Meal Preparation:
    - Plan and set up your feasts ahead of time to try not to depend on accommodation or quick food varieties.
    - This assists you with having command over fixings and piece sizes.

 Supplements:

- Think about supplements if necessary, like vitamin D, omega-3 unsaturated fats, or protein powder.
   - Talk with a medical services proficient or nutritionist prior to adding enhancements to your daily practice.

 Listen to Your Body:
   - Focus on what various food sources mean for your energy levels, absorption, and by and large prosperity.
   - Change your eating regimen in light of what cheers you up.

Moderation, Not Deprivation:
   - Permit yourself periodic treats with some restraint to keep a fair and maintainable methodology.
   - Prohibitive eating regimens are frequently more diligently to keep up with over the long haul.

 Consultation with a Nutritionist:
   - Consider looking for direction from an enlisted dietitian or nutritionist to fit your

nourishment plan to your particular requirements and objectives.

   - They can give customized counsel in view of elements like age, action level, and dietary inclinations.

Keep in mind, feasible changes in nourishment are a vital part of long haul progress in body change. It's about impermanent changes as well as embracing a solid and charming approach to eating that upholds your objectives.

Bodyweight exercises

Bodyweight rehearses are convincing for creating guts, determination, and flexibility without the prerequisite for additional equipment. Here is a once-over of bodyweight rehearses that target different muscle social occasions:

 Squats:
   - Targets: Quadriceps, hamstrings, glutes, and calves.
   - How: Stand with feet shoulder-width isolated, cut down your hips back and down, keeping your back straight, then, at that point, return to the starting position.

Lunges:
   - Targets: Quadriceps, hamstrings, glutes, and calves.

- How: Positive development with one foot, cut down your hips until the two knees are contorted at a 90-degree point, then, at that point, push back up to the starting position.

Push-Ups:
  - Targets: Chest, shoulders, back arm muscles, and focus.
  - How: Start in a board position, cut down your body by winding your elbows, then, push back up.

Pull-Ups (or Changed Rows):
  - Targets: Upper back, biceps, and shoulders.
  - How: Pull yourself up using a draw up bar or perform changed lines using an extreme even bar.

Planks:
  - Targets: Center muscles.
  - How: Start in a load up position, with your body in an efficient style from head to impact points, standing firm on the traction momentarily.

Burpees:

- Targets: Full-body work out, including cardiovascular diligence.
   - How: From a standing position, hunch down, kick your feet back into a board, play out a push-up, jump your feet back to your hands, and subsequently hazardously bounce up.

. **Mountain Climbers:**
   - Targets: Center, shoulders, and cardiovascular system.
   - How: Start in a board position, bring one knee toward your chest, then, switch legs rapidly in a running development.

Bodyweight Rows:
   - Targets: Upper back, biceps, and shoulders.
   - How: Use an extreme level bar at waist level, lie under it, and pull your chest up towards the bar.

 Dips:
   - Targets: Back arm muscles, shoulders, and chest.
   - How: Use equivalent bars or the edge of major areas of strength for a, cut down your

body by curving your elbows, then push back up.

 Hopping Jacks:
   - Targets: Cardiovascular system, legs, and shoulders.
   - How: Start with feet together, bob while spreading your arms and legs, then return to the starting position.

 Leg Raises:
   - Targets: Lower strong strength.
   - How: Lie on your back, raise your legs toward the rooftop, then lower them back down without permitting them to contact the ground.

Calf Raises:
   - Targets: Calves.
   - How: Stand on a level surface, raise your effect focuses by pushing through the pieces of your feet, then, lower them back down.

These exercises can be changed in accordance with various wellbeing levels and coordinated into a broad bodyweight rec center schedule ordinary practice. Persistently ensure authentic construction to increase practicality and reduce the bet of injury.

Outdoor and recreational activities

Taking part in open air and sporting exercises is a fabulous method for remaining dynamic and partake in the advantages of actual activity. Here are a few open air exercises that can add to your wellness process:

Hiking:
   - Investigate nature trails and climbing courses, appreciating both the actual work and the magnificence of the outside.

Cycling:
   - Ride a bicycle on trails or tourist detours, giving a great cardiovascular exercise while partaking in the natural air.

Running or Jogging:
   - Stir things up around town or run on nature trails to work on cardiovascular wellbeing and lift perseverance.

Swimming:
   - Exploit regular waterways or local area pools for a full-body exercise that is kind with the joints.

Kayaking or Canoeing:

- Paddle along streams or lakes to reinforce your chest area and center muscles.

 Rock Climbing:
   - Challenge yourself with rock climbing, whether at a climbing rec center or open air climbing regions.

Yoga in the Park:
   - Practice yoga outside to join the advantages of care and adaptability with the quieting impact of nature.

 Beach Volleyball:
   - Partake in a round of ocean side volleyball to connect with numerous muscle bunches while having a great time in the sun.

Stand-Up Paddleboarding (SUP):
   - Take a stab at paddleboarding on quiet waters to further develop balance and draw in your center muscles.

Outdoor Sports (Soccer, Baseball, etc.):
   - Arrange or join relaxed rounds of outside sports with companions to make wellness more friendly.

Gardening:
   - Digging, planting, and keeping a nursery can be an extraordinary low-influence active work that likewise gives a feeling of achievement.

Geocaching:
   - Consolidate open air investigation with treasure hunting by taking part in geocaching, a current expedition utilizing GPS facilitates.

Nature Walks:
   - Go for relaxed strolls in parks or nature holds, appreciating the landscape while remaining dynamic.

Outdoor Boot Camps:
   - Join or put together outside wellness classes or training camps that utilize regular components like seats, steps, and open spaces.

Golf:

- Partake in a series of golf, consolidating strolling and swinging for both active work and unwinding.

Keep in mind, the key is to track down exercises that you truly appreciate, making open air and sporting activities an essential and feasible piece of your wellness schedule. Whether alone or with companions, these exercises add to actual prosperity as well as give a reviving difference in view.

Mind-body connection

The psyche body association is a strong and unpredictable connection among mental and actual prosperity. Developing areas of strength for a body association can significantly affect generally wellbeing. Here are key viewpoints and practices to consider:

Mindfulness and Meditation:
   - Practice care and contemplation to carry attention to the current second.
   - These practices upgrade mindfulness and encourage a more profound association between the psyche and body.

Breathing Exercises:
   - Center around controlled breathing procedures to lessen pressure and advance unwinding.

- Profound, deliberate breaths can decidedly impact both mental and actual states.

Yoga and Tai Chi:
   - Take part in rehearses like yoga or jujitsu that join actual development with breath and care.
   - These exercises advance adaptability, balance, and an agreeable association between the brain and body.

Visualization:
   - Use perception methods to envision positive results, which can emphatically affect actual execution and prosperity.

Positive Affirmations:
   - Develop a positive outlook through insistences.
   - Positive self-talk can impact certainty, inspiration, and the body's reaction to push.

 Stress Management:
   - Foster powerful pressure the executives procedures, for example, recognizing stressors and tracking down solid survival techniques.

- Ongoing pressure can adversely influence both mental and actual wellbeing.

Biofeedback:
- Investigate biofeedback methods that give constant data about physiological reactions (pulse, muscle strain).
- This mindfulness can support directing these reactions through mental concentration.

Holistic Wellbeing Practices:
- Consider comprehensive wellbeing rehearses like needle therapy, back rub, or chiropractic care.
- These practices mean to adjust energy stream and upgrade the body's normal abilities to mend.

Physical Action as Self-Care:
- View actual work not just for the purpose of working on actual wellbeing yet additionally as a type of taking care of oneself for mental prosperity.

Journaling:

- Keep a diary to offer viewpoints and feelings.
- Thinking about encounters can extend understanding and fortify the brain body association.

 Gratitude Practice:
- Develop an appreciation practice by zeroing in on sure parts of life.
- Appreciation has been connected to worked on mental and actual wellbeing.

Listening to Body Signals:
- Focus on actual sensations and signs from the body.
- Tuning into yearning, weakness, and different sensations encourages a superior comprehension of your body's requirements.

Cognitive Conduct Treatment (CBT):
- Consider CBT methods to address and reexamine negative idea designs.
- This can emphatically influence close to home prosperity and, hence, actual wellbeing.

Laughter and Joy:

- Consolidate exercises that give pleasure and giggling.

- Chuckling triggers the arrival of endorphins, adding to a positive brain body association.

By effectively sustaining the brain body association, people can encounter a more incorporated and all encompassing way to deal with wellbeing. The collaboration among mental and actual prosperity is a powerful relationship that, when sustained, adds to generally flexibility and imperativeness.

Recovery and rest

Recuperation and rest are vital parts of any successful wellness or health schedule. Here are key contemplations for streamlining recuperation and guaranteeing satisfactory rest:

Sleep Quality:
   - Focus on adequate and quality rest to help physical and mental recuperation.
   - Go for the gold long stretches of rest each evening, as rest is fundamental for muscle fix and in general prosperity.

 Active Recovery:
   - Integrate light, low-influence exercises on rest days to improve blood dissemination and advance adaptability.
   - Exercises like strolling, swimming, or delicate yoga can be advantageous.

 Hydration:

- Remain all around hydrated to help the body's normal recuperation processes.
   - Water supports supplement transport and helps flush out metabolic side-effects from work out.

Nutrition for Recovery:
   - Consume a fair post-practice dinner or tidbit that incorporates protein and starches.
   - Supplement thick food varieties support muscle recuperation and renew glycogen stores.

Foam Rolling and Stretching:
   - Use froth rollers or take part in extending schedules to lighten muscle snugness and upgrade adaptability.
   - Target areas of irritation or strain to work on by and large portability.

 Rest Days:
   - Plan customary rest days inside your gym routine daily schedule to forestall overtraining.
   - Rest days permit muscles and the focal sensory system to recuperate and adjust.

Mindfulness and Unwinding Techniques:
   - Practice care or unwinding strategies, like profound breathing or contemplation, to oversee pressure and advance mental recuperation.

Massage or Bodywork:
   - Consider normal back rubs or other bodywork treatments to decrease muscle strain and upgrade recuperation.
   - These practices can likewise further develop course and adaptability.

Heat and Cold Therapy:
   - Use heat treatment (hot showers or warming cushions) or cold treatment (ice packs) to oversee irritation and lessen muscle irritation.

Listen to Your Body:
   - Focus on signs of weariness, touchiness, or diminished execution.
   - Change your exercise force or accept extra rest depending on the situation.

Sleep Environment:

- Establish a helpful rest climate with an agreeable sleeping pad, cushions, and a cool, dull room.
    - Guarantee your rest climate upholds helpful rest.

 Consistent Rest Schedule:
    - Lay out a steady rest plan by hitting the hay and awakening simultaneously every day.
    - This controls the body's interior clock for better rest quality.

Hormonal Balance:
    - Be aware of hormonal irregular characteristics that might influence recuperation, particularly for ladies.
    - Factors, for example, monthly cycle stages can impact energy levels and exercise execution.

Recovery Tools:
    - Consider utilizing recuperation devices like pressure articles of clothing, Epsom salt showers, or even cryotherapy to support muscle recuperation.

Offsetting active work with satisfactory recuperation is fundamental for upgrading execution, forestalling wounds, and advancing by and large prosperity. Tailor your recuperation techniques to accommodate your singular necessities and pay attention to your body's signs for rest and revival.

Technology and fitness apps

Incorporating innovation and wellness applications into your routine can upgrade your general wellbeing and assist you with accomplishing your wellness objectives. Here are far to use innovation for a more powerful and pleasant wellness experience:

Fitness Following Apps:
   - Put applications like MyFitnessPal to good use or It will quit being useful! to follow your everyday nourishment and screen your calorie consumption.
   - Wellness trackers, for example, Fitbit or Apple Watch can screen your everyday movement levels, pulse, and rest designs.

Workout Apps:

- Investigate exercise applications like Nike Preparing Club, FitOn, or Brief Exercise for directed work-out schedules customized to your wellness level and objectives.
- Yoga applications like Yoga for Amateurs or Day to day Yoga can direct you through different stances and schedules.

Personalized Preparing Programs:
- Consider applications that deal customized preparing programs in view of your wellness objectives, like Freeletics or JEFIT.
- These applications frequently adjust exercises to your advancement and inclinations.

Running and Cycling Apps:
- Applications like Strava or MapMyRun can follow your running or cycling courses, give continuous information, and proposition a local area for sharing accomplishments.
- Virtual cycling applications like Zwift add an intelligent component to indoor cycling.

Virtual Classes and Web based Services:

- Partake in virtual wellness classes through stages like Peloton, which offers a scope of exercises from cycling to strength preparing.
- Web-based features like YouTube or particular wellness applications frequently highlight an assortment of exercise routine schedules drove by wellness experts.

Wearable Wellness Technology:
- Put resources into wearable gadgets like smartwatches or wellness trackers for ongoing observing of your actual work, pulse, and rest.
- These gadgets can give bits of knowledge into your general wellbeing and energize a more dynamic way of life.

Nutrition Apps:
- Investigate nourishment applications like Yazio or MyPlate to log your dinners, track macronutrients, and get customized sustenance exhortation.
- Food conveyance applications with solid choices can work on feast arranging.

Mindfulness and Contemplation Apps:

- Use care and contemplation applications like Headspace or Quiet to oversee pressure, further develop concentration, and improve generally prosperity.
   - A large number of these applications offer fast, directed meetings that can be effortlessly coordinated into your day to day daily schedule.

Social Wellness Platforms:
   - Join wellness networks on friendly stages or applications, interfacing with similar people for inspiration and backing.
   - Stages like Fitbit and Strava have local area includes that permit you to share accomplishments and draw in with others.

AR and VR Fitness:
   - Investigate increased reality (AR) or augmented reality (VR) wellness applications that give vivid exercise encounters.
   - Applications like Powerful for VR or AR exercises can make practice really captivating.

Smart Home Wellness Equipment:
   - Put resources into brilliant home wellness hardware, similar to savvy treadmills or

exercise bikes, that can adjust with applications and give intuitive exercise encounters.

Incorporating innovation into your wellness routine can change it up, inspiration, and comfort. Pick applications and gadgets that line up with your objectives and inclinations, making your wellness process more customized and pleasant.

Adapting to lifestyle changes

Adjusting to way of life changes is fundamental for keeping an economical and sound wellness venture. Here are down to earth procedures to help you embrace and effectively coordinate way of life changes:

Start Small:
   - Start with sensible changes to try not to feel overpowered.

- Progressively expand on these progressions as they become piece of your daily schedule.

Set Sensible Goals:
   - Characterize clear, attainable objectives that line up with your way of life and needs.
   - Break bigger objectives into more modest, feasible achievements for a feeling of achievement.

 Prioritize Consistency:
   - Center around consistency instead of flawlessness.
   - Little, steady endeavors after some time lead to additional feasible outcomes.

Establish Routine:
   - Make an everyday or week by week schedule that integrates wellness and health exercises.
   - Consistency helps structure propensities that become imbued in your way of life.

Time Management:
   - Focus on and plan time for active work inside your everyday daily practice.
   - Treat it as a fundamental piece of your timetable, very much like different responsibilities.

Incorporate Action into Day to day Life:
   - Search for amazing chances to be dynamic over the course of the

day, like using the stairwell, strolling, or extending during breaks.
   - Transform day to day assignments into open doors for development.

Find Agreeable Activities:
   - Pick proactive tasks that you truly appreciate.
   - Whether it's moving, climbing, or playing a game, delight improves the probability of long haul responsibility.

Adapt Exercises to Your Schedule:
   - Select exercise routine schedules that fit your time imperatives.

- Short, focused energy exercises can be essentially as successful as longer meetings.

Meal Arranging and Prep:
- Plan and get ready feasts ahead of time to guarantee admittance to nutritious choices.
- Group cooking can save time and advance smart dieting.

Stay Flexible:
- Be adaptable and adjust your wellness routine to changes in your timetable or surprising occasions.
- Acknowledge that a few days might include changes to your arrangement.

Seek Support:

- Share your wellness objectives with companions, family, or an exercise pal.
    - Having an emotionally supportive network can give consolation and responsibility.

Celebrate Progress:
    - Recognize and commend your accomplishments, regardless of how little.
    - Encouraging feedback improves inspiration and supports force.

Reflect and Adjust:
    - Consistently survey your advancement and rethink your objectives.
    - Change your methodology in light of what turns out best for you.

Embrace a Development Mindset:
   - Embrace a development outlook that perspectives challenges as any open doors for learning and improvement.
   - Embrace the excursion of self-awareness.

Mind-Body Integration:
   - Perceive the interconnectedness of physical and mental prosperity.
   - Focus on exercises that advance both physical and psychological well-being.

Adjusting to way of life changes is a continuous interaction that requires persistence and self-empathy. By causing changes that to line up with your extraordinary conditions and inclinations, you can make a way of life that upholds your general wellbeing and prosperity.

Tracking progress

Following headway is essential for remaining roused and making informed acclimations to your wellness process. Here are successful ways of checking and measure your advancement:

Set Clear Goals:
  - Characterize explicit and quantifiable objectives that line up with your general wellness targets.
  - Whether it's weight reduction, strength gains, or further developed perseverance, lucidity is critical.

Keep an Exercise Journal:
  - Record your exercises, including works out, sets, reps, and any notes about how you felt during the meeting.

- Following your exercises recognizes examples and regions for development.

Use Wellness Apps:
   - Use wellness applications or wearables to follow different measurements, for example, steps taken, calories consumed, and exercise power.
   - Numerous applications likewise permit you to log sustenance and screen progress over the long haul.

Take Customary Measurements:
   - Track changes in your body estimations, like abdomen outline, hips, chest, and other pertinent regions.
   - These estimations can give a more extensive perspective on your advancement.

Capture Progress Photos:
   - Routinely take photographs to report your actual changes outwardly.
   - Contrasting pictures after some time can be a strong inspiration.

Monitor Strength and Performance:

- Track your solidarity levels by recording the loads, reps, and sets for each activity.
   - Expanding strength is a substantial indication of progress.

Assess Cardiovascular Fitness:
   - Assess cardiovascular advancement by checking factors like running velocity, cycling distance, or the time it takes to finish explicit exercises.
   - Progressive upgrades demonstrate improved perseverance.

Measure Adaptability and Mobility:
   - Evaluate changes in adaptability and versatility through practices like extending or yoga.
   - Further developed scope of movement is a positive pointer.

Keep a Nourishment Log:
   - Log your everyday food admission to screen dietary propensities.
   - Understanding what your eating regimen means for your objectives is fundamental for supported progress.

Track Rest and Recovery:
   - Focus on your rest examples and how well you recuperate between exercises.
   - Quality rest is significant for ideal execution and recuperation.

 Regular Check-Ins:
   - Plan customary registrations with yourself to think about your advancement.
   - Celebrate accomplishments and reevaluate objectives if important.

 Use Benchmark Workouts:
   - Consolidate benchmark exercises or wellness evaluations at standard spans.
   - These can act as reference focuses for development.

Celebrate Non-Scale Victories:
   - Recognize and celebrate non-scale triumphs, for example, further developed mind-set, expanded energy levels, or improved mental concentration.
   - Positive changes stretch out past actual estimations.

Consider Body Creation Analysis:
   - Investigate strategies like muscle versus fat ratio estimations to acquire bits of knowledge into changes in muscle and fat conveyance.
   - Some wellness trackers or expert appraisals can give this data.

 Seek Proficient Guidance:
   - Talk with wellness experts or medical services suppliers for occasional evaluations.
   - They can give master experiences and proposals in light of your advancement.

Consistently assessing and investigating your advancement guarantees that your wellness process stays dynamic and custom fitted to your developing objectives. Utilize a blend of genuine estimations and emotional perceptions to make a complete perspective on your accomplishments and regions for development.

Overcoming challenges

Beating difficulties is an innate piece of any wellness venture. Here are procedures to help you explore and vanquish normal snags on your way to accomplishing your wellbeing and health objectives:

Set Sensible Expectations:
   - Lay out attainable and practical objectives to try not to get yourself in a position for superfluous difficulties.
   - Perceive that progress requires some investment.

 Develop a Development Mindset:
   - Develop a development mentality that perspectives challenges as any open doors for learning and improvement.

- Embrace mishaps as a characteristic piece of the excursion.

Break Objectives into More modest Steps:
   - Partition bigger objectives into more modest, more reasonable advances.
   - Accomplishing these more modest achievements assembles certainty and inspiration.

Create a Help System:
   - Construct an encouraging group of people with companions, family, or exercise pals.
   - Share your objectives and difficulties, and look for support during troublesome times.

Adaptability:
   - Be adaptable and able to adjust your methodology as conditions change.
   - Change your objectives and procedures to suit what is going on.

Learn from Setbacks:
   - View difficulties as any open doors to learn and develop.

- Distinguish the elements adding to difficulties and use them as experiences for development.

Problem-Addressing Skills:
- Foster critical thinking abilities to explore unforeseen obstructions.
- Track down effective fixes to address difficulties that emerge.

Consistent Effort:
- Focus on consistency over flawlessness.
- Reliable exertion, in any event, when confronted with difficulties, adds to long haul achievement.

Mindfulness and Stress Management:
- Practice care and stress the board methods to adapt to difficulties.
- Strategies like profound breathing or reflection can assist you with keeping on track and tough.

Celebrate Little Wins:
- Recognize and celebrate little triumphs en route.

- Perceiving progress, regardless of how minor, supports inspiration.

Adjust Objectives as Needed:
- Rethink and change your objectives in light of evolving conditions.
- Adjust your assumptions to line up with your ongoing reality.

Seek Proficient Guidance:
- Talk with wellness experts, nutritionists, or psychological well-being specialists when confronted with explicit difficulties.
- Proficient direction can give custom-made arrangements and backing.

Positive Self-Talk:
- Develop positive self-converse with counter regrettable contemplations during testing times.
- Supplant self-uncertainty with certifications and a faith in your capacity to beat deterrents.

Stay Focused on the Process:
- Help yourself to remember the reasons you left on your wellness process.

- Remain focused on the interaction, in any event, when confronted with troubles.

Learn to Oversee Time Effectively:
- Focus on using time effectively to offset wellness endeavors with different responsibilities.
- Plan and timetable your exercises and taking care of oneself exercises.

Keep in mind, challenges are a characteristic piece of any groundbreaking excursion. By embracing a versatile outlook, looking for help, and constantly adjusting, you can beat impediments and arise more grounded on your way to accomplishing your wellbeing and health objectives.